CANKER SORES

Mouth Ulcer Healing: Help for Those Who Have Canker Sores

CARL JUAN

Table of Contents

Introductory

Aphthous ulcers, more often known as canker sores, are small, painful sores that can appear on the gums, inner cheeks, tongue, and roof of the mouth. Cold sores, which are also caused by the herpes virus but more commonly appear on the lips or outside of the mouth, are not the same thing.

• Canker sores typically have a red border and a round or oval shape. They come in a wide range of sizes and can cause a lot of discomfort, especially while trying to eat or talk. Canker sores can have a number of different causes, and it's not always possible to pinpoint the precise one.

• Accidental biting or braces irritation are two common causes of mild oral damage.

• Emotional strain or stress.

• Hormonal shifts.

• Intolerances or allergies to certain foods.

• Damage to the body's defenses.

• Some fundamental health problems.

• Canker sores seldom cause any serious complications and typically heal on their own within a week or two. Though painful, they can be alleviated with over-the-counter or prescribed topical pain relievers or pharmaceuticals. Canker sores that recur frequently, are unusually large or chronic, or are accompanied by other troubling symptoms should prompt a trip to the doctor for diagnosis and possible treatment.

CHAPTER ONE
Canker Sore Subtypes

Depending on the severity, frequency, and etiology, canker sores fall into one of three broad categories:

• The most prevalent form of canker sores is the minor variety. They rarely leave scars and often heal after a week or two; their average diameter is less than a third of an inch (7 mm).

• Canker sores of the major variety are bigger and more painful than the more common minor variety. They can be beyond 1/3 inch (7 mm) in diameter and may take many weeks to recover. Canker sores, if they get severe enough, can leave scars.

• Herpetiform canker sores are the rarest form of this condition. Clusters of several small sores that eventually combine into larger, oddly shaped ulcers are a hallmark of this condition. Despite their name, they are not linked to the herpes virus.

Canker sores have a complex etiology that may differ from person to person. Canker sores can be caused by a number of different things, including stress, hormonal shifts, dietary sensitivities or allergies, a compromised immune system, and even some diseases. Canker sores are not the same thing as cold sores, which are caused by the herpes simplex virus and often show up on or near the lips.

Most Typical Signs

Signs of an aphthous ulcer, often known as a canker sore, include:

• Canker sores can be rather painful, especially in their early stages of growth and when they initially appear. Pain can make even simple activities like eating or drinking unpleasant.

- **Discomfort:** Even when not actively suffering intense pain, canker sores can cause a general discomfort or irritation in the mouth.

- Canker sores, as lesions go, are often spherical or oval in shape, with a red border and a white or yellowish center. They seem different from other types of mouth sores and are easily identifiable as such.

- Their typical habitat is the mouth's soft tissues, including the gums, inside cheeks, tongue, and roof. The throat and tonsils are less common sites for these growths.

- Canker sores range in size from little larger than a pinhead to around the diameter of a small coin.

- Canker sores have an average healing time of two weeks when left untreated. Formation, growth, and repair are some of the possible stages of development.

It's vital to highlight that canker sores are not connected with fever or other systemic symptoms. Although they may cause some discomfort, they pose no serious health risks. If you have a history of frequent and severe canker sores, or if you develop canker sores that are unusually large, persistent, or accompanied by other concerning symptoms, it is best to see a doctor to rule out any underlying medical conditions and to receive treatment or management strategies.

CHAPTER TWO
Canker Sore Origins

Aphthous ulcers, more often known as canker sores, can have a number of different causes. Canker sores have many potential causes and contributors, including:

• **Minor Mouth Injuries:** Trauma to the mouth, such as accidently biting the inside of your cheek or tongue, using abrasive dental care products, or injury from dental procedures, can cause the growth of canker sores.

• Emotional and psychological factors include stress and anxiety, both of which can suppress the immune system and contribute to the onset of canker sores.

• Canker sores may be more common in people whose hormone levels fluctuate often, as may happen during pregnancy, menopause, or menstruation.

• Canker sores can appear in the mouth when the sensitive tissues are irritated, as can happen when eating foods that are too acidic or too hot. Canker sores have been linked to gluten intolerance and other food sensitivities.

• Canker sores are more common in those who have a compromised immune system as a result of sickness, treatment, or underlying medical disorders.

• Canker sore susceptibility may be influenced by one's genetic make-up. Canker sores are more common in people who have a family history of the condition.

• The development of canker sores has been linked to a number of different viruses. Although this does happen occasionally, it is much less prevalent than with cold sores, which are caused by the herpes simplex virus.

- **Certain Medical Conditions:** Conditions such as inflammatory bowel disease, celiac disease, Behçet's disease, and HIV/AIDS have been related with an increased risk of canker sores.

Canker sores are not communicable and typically have a benign course. They are a fairly typical oral health problem and usually clear up on their own within a week or two. However, they often hurt and are otherwise unpleasant. Medications and topical treatments, both over-the-counter and prescribed, may alleviate symptoms and speed recovery. Canker sores can be a symptom of a number of different conditions, so it's important to see a doctor if you have them frequently, if they're unusually large or persistent, or if they're accompanied by other worrying symptoms.

Keeping Canker Sores at Bay

It may be difficult to completely avoid getting canker sores, also known as aphthous ulcers, but there are measures you can do to lessen their likelihood and impact.

1. Take Care of Your Teeth:

• If you suffer from oral sensitivity, try using a toothpaste without sodium lauryl sulfate (SLS) and a soft-bristled toothbrush.

• If you want to avoid canker sores, it's important to keep your mouth clean and clear of food particles by flossing every day.

2. Take Care with Your Food Choices:

• Stay away from spicy, acidic, or salty foods because these can aggravate canker sores in certain people.

• If you have canker sores and think certain foods may be the cause, cutting them out of your diet may help.

3. Tension Control:

• Stress is a common trigger for canker sores. Take slow breaths, meditate, do yoga, or go for a run if you're feeling overwhelmed.

• Strive for a good work-life balance and make sure you're getting enough sleep.

4. When you eat and chew, be careful not to bite your tongue or cheek.

• Do not use mouthwashes or toothpastes that are too harsh on your teeth.

5. Hormonal Stability:

• If you have recurring canker sores around the time of your period, you may want to discuss hormone management measures with your doctor.

6. Supplementing with vitamin B complex, folic acid, or iron has helped some persons with canker sores. Consult with a healthcare physician before starting any new supplements.

7. Take Care of Your Root Health Issues

• Canker sores may be less common if you have a medical condition like celiac disease or inflammatory bowel disease that is under control.

8. Keep up with Good Oral Hygiene:

• Canker sores may be caused by tooth problems, thus it's important to have regular dental checkups.

9. Medically-Preferred Drugs:

• Prescription drugs, such as topical corticosteroids or antibacterial mouthwashes, may be recommended by a healthcare provider to treat canker sores.

10. Testing for Allergies:

• See an allergist for evaluation and advice if you have canker sores and think allergies may be to blame.

Keep in mind that these preventative measures can have varying degrees of success depending on the person, and that what works for one person may not work for another. Canker sores can be a symptom of a number of different conditions, so it's important to see a doctor if you have them frequently, if they're unusually large or persistent, or if they're accompanied by other worrying symptoms.

CHAPTER THREE
Canker Sore Treatments At Home

Canker sores are painful and annoying, but there are a few things you can do at home that might make you feel better and speed up the healing process. Canker sore treatments at home include:

• Warm salt water gargling or rinsing can alleviate discomfort and speed healing. Swish a glass of warm water containing half a teaspoon of salt for 30 seconds before spitting it out.

2. Sodium bicarbonate paste:

• Baking soda and a tiny bit of water can be made into a paste. Apply the paste directly to the canker sore, leave it on for a few minutes, and then rinse your mouth. The soreness may be relieved by this.

3. Honey:

• If you get a canker sore, try dabbing some honey on it. Honey's antibacterial and analgesic characteristics make it a popular natural remedy.

4. Extract from Coconuts:

• Coconut oil can reduce inflammation and kill bacteria. Coconut oil can be applied directly to the canker sore to alleviate discomfort and swelling.

5. Gel from the Aloe Vera Plant:

• Because of its calming effects, aloe vera gel is widely used. If you have a canker sore, try applying some aloe vera gel straight to the sore.

6. Magnesium milk:

• A canker sore's acidity can be neutralized and irritation lessened by applying a little dab of milk of magnesia.

7. To shave or not to shave:

• Numb the area and lower discomfort and swelling by letting ice melt in your mouth or sucking on ice chips.

8. Root Extract of Liquorice:

• You can use a gel or paste made from licorice root extract directly to the canker sore to relieve discomfort and speed healing.

9. Antioxidant Oil, or Vitamin E:

• Break open a pill of vitamin E and dab the oil on the canker sore. The recovery time may be shortened because of this.

10. A Cup of Chamomile:

• Brew a chamomile tea bag, let it cool, and use it as a mouthwash to treat canker sores.

11. OTC Lotions, Creams, and Lotions:

• Canker sore treatment over-the-counter (OTC) medications are available at most pharmacies. These may contain anesthetics and healing agents like benzocaine and hydrogen peroxide.

12. Eating Sensitive Foods:

• Canker sores can heal more slowly if you eat spicy, acidic, or salty foods, so it's best to steer clear of these.

Although these home treatments can be helpful, not everyone will have the same experience with them. Canker sores that are very large, chronic, or accompanied by other worrying symptoms warrant a trip to the doctor for a thorough evaluation and diagnosis to rule out more serious illnesses.

Seeking the Advice of Experts

You should consult a doctor or dentist if you have canker sores that are particularly large, persistent, or accompanied by other worrying symptoms, or if you have them repeatedly. If you have canker sores, you should see a doctor because...

• Canker sores should be taken seriously, and medical attention sought, if they occur frequently (more than a few times a year), or if they are very large, painful, or long-lasting.

• Underlying Medical Conditions:
If you feel that an underlying
medical condition may be
contributing to the canker sores,
such as celiac disease, inflammatory
bowel disease, or an immune
system disorder, obtaining medical
assessment and testing is
necessary.

• Consult a medical practitioner to
rule out more serious problems if
your canker sores are accompanied
by other odd or alarming symptoms
such as high fever, exhaustion, joint
pain, or widespread oral lesions.

• If canker sores are making it
painful or impossible for you to eat,

drink, or otherwise use your mouth normally, medical attention is warranted.

• If you have tried over-the-counter medications and home therapies without success, it may be time to see a doctor or dentist who can prescribe stronger medication or suggest other courses of therapy.

• Children's mouth sores: see a pediatrician or dentist for advice if the canker sores come back frequently or are severe.

If you have canker sores, it's best to see a doctor so they can examine you, determine what's causing them, and give you advice on how to cure or manage them. This may involve prescription drugs, oral rinses, or other interventions to assist ease the pain and encourage healing.

Keep in mind that canker sores, despite being painful and annoying, are mostly harmless and not contagious. If your canker sores are causing you concern or if they are severely limiting your everyday activities, it is essential that you get professional assistance.

CHAPTER FOUR
Therapeutic Interventions

When canker sores (aphthous ulcers) become severe, persistent, or unresponsive to self-care measures, medical intervention may be necessary. Your doctor or dentist may suggest the following procedures for you:

1. Creams and Lotions:

• To alleviate discomfort and speed healing, canker sores may be treated topically. Some of these are:

To numb the area and alleviate discomfort, you can use over-the-counter or prescribed oral gels or ointments containing chemicals like benzocaine.

• Ointments and lotions containing corticosteroids, available with a doctor's prescription, can help reduce inflammation and hasten the healing process. Those are reserved for canker sores that are particularly large or painful.

2. Drugs taken via mouth:

• If your canker sores are exceptionally severe or are related to another medical issue, your doctor may recommend oral treatments.

In severe cases, your doctor may recommend taking corticosteroid medications to lessen inflammation and pain.

• Oral Antiseptics: Prescription antimicrobial or antiseptic rinses or drugs can help reduce inflammation and prevent secondary bacterial infections.

3. Vitamins and Minerals:

• Your doctor may suggest taking a supplement containing vitamin B12, folic acid, or iron if he or she suspects that your canker sores are caused by a nutrient deficiency.

4. Treatment with a Cautery or Laser:

- Sometimes dentists and other medical professionals will cauterize (burn) a canker sore to close the wound and alleviate the pain. To alleviate discomfort and speed recovery, laser therapy may be utilized instead.

5. Oral Hygiene:

- Hydrogen peroxide and other antiseptic chemicals may be included in the list of recommended mouthwashes and rinses from your doctor.

6. Prescription Drugs for Chronic Illnesses:

• If an underlying medical condition is leading to canker sores, treating that disease may help avoid the recurrence of sores.

7. Injections of Steroids into the Joint:

• Your doctor may choose to inject corticosteroids right into the canker sore if it is exceedingly painful or resistant to other treatments.

8. Drugs That Alter the Immune System: Canker sores that are particularly painful or persistent may require immunomodulatory treatments such thalidomide or colchicine, albeit they have serious adverse effects and should be used only as a last resort.

The best course of action depends on your unique condition; therefore it's important to talk to your doctor or dentist about it. They can give an accurate diagnosis, uncover any underlying reasons, and recommend the most effective therapies to manage the discomfort and encourage healing of your canker sores.

Treating Canker Sores

Canker sores are annoying and painful, making it difficult to deal with them. Managing and coping with canker sores can be done with the following methods:

1. Drugs Available Without a Prescription: Numb the sore and relieve discomfort with over-the-counter topical gels or ointments containing chemicals like benzocaine.

Antimicrobial mouth rinses are available without a prescription and may be used to lessen the likelihood of infection.

2. Medically-Preferred Drugs:

• Prescription drugs, such as topical corticosteroids or oral medications, may be prescribed to ease pain and promote healing if your canker sores are severe, persistent, or do not respond to over-the-counter therapies.

3. Reduced Pain:

• To alleviate pain and discomfort, try taking an over-the-counter pain medicine such ibuprofen or acetaminophen. Always use the prescribed amount.

4. Eating Sensitive Foods:

• Avoid foods that are hot, acidic, or salty since they may irritate the canker sores.

• Go for bland, soft foods, and try to eat healthily overall.

5. Personal Oral Hygiene:

• Keep your mouth healthy by using a soft-bristled toothbrush to gently clean your teeth twice a day and by flossing regularly to remove food particles stuck between your teeth and avoid infection and inflammation.

6. Creams and Lotions:

• Canker sores can be relieved with a saltwater rinse, a paste made of baking soda, honey, coconut oil, or aloe vera gel.

7. Ice:

• Numb the area and lower discomfort and swelling by letting ice melt in your mouth or sucking on ice chips.

8. Reducing Stress:

• Emotional tension, which can lead to canker sores, can be managed by relaxation techniques like deep breathing, meditation, or yoga.

9. Measures for Safety:

• Biting your cheeks or lips can lead to canker sores, so it's best to refrain from doing so.

• If your braces or dentures are causing you discomfort, talk to your dentist or orthodontist about getting them adjusted.

10. Don't drink or smoke:

• Tobacco and alcohol are both known to irritate the mouth, which can make canker sores worse. Consider limiting or eliminating these chemicals.

11. Spit Out After Eating:

• After eating, give your mouth a soft rinsing with water to get rid of any leftover food particles that could irritate the sores.

12. Maintain a Food Journal:

• Keeping a food diary will help you figure out which foods may be causing your canker sores.

13. Seek the Advice of a Medical Professional:

• If your canker sores are frequent, severe, or accompanied by uncommon symptoms, consult a healthcare physician or dentist for a proper diagnosis and treatment suggestions.

14. Mutual Aid Societies

• Canker sore sufferers can benefit from connecting with others who share their condition by joining in-person or virtual support groups.

Keep in mind that canker sores, despite being unpleasant, are harmless, and usually disappear on their own. Canker sores often heal within a week to a fortnight. It is important to see a doctor if your canker sores are giving you substantial discomfort or interfering with your regular life.

Conclusion

Canker sores, also called aphthous ulcers, are painful ulcers that form on the interior of the mouth and are quite frequent. They may be irritating, but fever blisters seldom cause any harm and often heal on their own within a week or two at most. Minor oral injuries, stress, hormonal shifts, dietary sensitivities, a weaker immune system, and underlying medical disorders are just some of the many potential causes of canker sores.

Canker sores are treated with a combination of home remedies and, in severe situations, medical intervention. Some effective home remedies for pain and inflammation include ice, honey, baking soda pastes, and saltwater rinses. More severe or persistent canker sores may benefit from topical and oral drugs available over-the-counter or on prescription.

Large, chronic canker sores, especially if accompanied by other symptoms, warrant a visit to the dentist or doctor. They will be able to properly diagnose your canker sores, advise you on the best course of treatment, and aid you in coping with the pain you experience.

Canker sores, while annoying, can be managed to the point that they have no effect on everyday life and recover within a reasonable amount of time.

THE END